Writing a
History
&
Physical

Writing a History & Physical

Jeffrey L. Greenwald, MD
Assistant Professor of Medicine
Boston University School of Medicine
Boston Medical Center
Boston, Massachusetts

HANLEY & BELFUS
An imprint of Elsevier

HANLEY & BELFUS

An Imprint of Elsevier
*

The Curtis Center
Independence Square West
Philadelphia, Pennsylvania 19107

Library of Congress Control Number: 2003101350

WRITING A HISTORY AND PHYSICAL   ISBN 1-56053-602-0

Transferred to Digital Printing 2009

Contents

Preface

Learning the process of writing an effective history and physical (H&P) is a major hurdle for trainees. Despite the fact that good written communications skills are clearly a critical part of patient care, they do not always receive the emphasis in training that they require. To complicate this problem, trainees often perceive that their preceptors want differing elements in the write-up and in different orders. There are many variations in style and format to confuse the new trainee.

This guide takes the learner, whether he or she is a medical, nursing, nurse practitioner, or physician assistant trainee, through the major steps of the process of writing a complete, thoughtful, and well-developed H&P. As such, the guide explains the **purpose of each step, not simply the content.** Therefore, no matter what the "local culture" is of the service on which the trainee is working, he or she will understand **why certain elements of the H&P go where they go** and **what each section of the H&P must accomplish** to permit excellence in communications and patient care.

Remember, learning how to write an H&P is a process. It takes time, experience, careful consideration, and a willingness to seek out critique. In the end, however, the mastery of—or at least competency in—the process will serve the trainee and his or her patients well.

Jeffrey L. Greenwald, MD

The Abridged Guide to Writing a History and Physical

Source
- Very brief
- Identify the source(s) of information
- Comment on the credibility of the source

Chief Complaint
- Brief statement of why the patient presented
- Identifies patient and relevant "context" related to presenting complaint
- Focuses attention of reader

History of Present Illness (HPI)
- Lead the reader toward the conclusions you draw in the Assessment and Plan that follows.
- Write in full sentences.
- Do not make up abbreviations.
- Organize and edit the patient's information.
- Give the time course.
- Be descriptive, not analytic, regarding all features of the primary complaint(s).
- Include all relevant information about the complaint(s).
- Note other coexisting illnesses/situations that may contribute ("context").
- Guide the reader through the appropriate differential diagnosis with pertinent positives and negatives.

Past Medical History (PMH)
- Thorough listing of prior medical illnesses or events

- Include supporting data (e.g., biopsies, PFTs, echos, CTs, if available)
- Avoid chart lore
- Consider separating past surgical, obstetric, and psychiatric histories

Meds
- List all meds, doses, routes, intervals
- Include over-the-counter meds
- Include recently stopped or changed meds

Allergies
- List all meds to which patient has reacted
- List the reaction

Family History
- List or diagram family members
- List major illness, causes of death for each family member

Social History
- Occupation, hobbies, personal interests
- Marital status, number of children, social support network, living situation
- Alcohol, cigarette, and illicit drug use
- Sexual history
- May choose to split this into: Social History, Occupational History, and Habits

Review of Systems
- Comprehensive head-to-toe or system-by-system checklist of symptoms
- If relevant (positive or negative) to HPI, it belongs in HPI—not here

■ Any significant findings require follow-up in Assessment and Plan sections below

Physical Exam
■ Describe, don't interpret, findings
■ Be systematic—e.g., General Appearance, Vitals, HEENT, Neck, Lungs, Cardiac, Breast, Abdomen, Rectum, Genitals, Extremities, Skin, Musculoskeletal, Neuro

Labs/Data
■ Common labs first (CBC, chemistries, liver functions, coagulation profile)
■ Other blood tests obtained
■ Urinalysis
■ Chest x-ray (and other radiology studies)
■ ECG
■ Other data obtained

Assessment
■ Demonstrate your thinking process.
■ Don't summarize; *synthesize.*
■ Include key elements of H&P in a guided fashion to lead the reader through the differential diagnosis and land the reader on your conclusion(s).
■ Generate a problem list (primary and secondary) with explanations considering why and how this situation occurred.
■ Write in full sentences.

Plan
■ This may be integrated into Assessment section.
■ Enumerate a specific problem list as above.

- Be as specific with your plans as possible.
- Address all issues.

Writing a History and Physical

What follows is a tool for approaching a very difficult aspect of being a member of a medical team: **how to write a *comprehensive, clear,* and most importantly *useful* admission history and physical**—hereafter referred to as the H&P. As you will discover, writing the H&P is probably as much art as science, and as such, many different versions will be used by different doctors. The goals of all the differing styles are the same:

1. Communicating the important aspects of the patient's presentation
2. Providing thorough background information about the patient
3. Leading the reader through the information in an organized manner so he or she can understand what you were thinking when you made treatment decisions

These may seem intuitive, but putting them into practice is not always so easy. Let's touch on each of them briefly for further explanation.

✓ *Communicating the important aspects of the patient's presentation*

Think about this aspect of the H&P as if you were building a house. The materials (i.e., information you need) for the house may come from different suppliers (different sources such as the patient, the family, the primary care physician, old records) and **you will have to re-organize (edit) them** before you actually start the construction. You also need to make sure that you have all the parts (or information) you will need for the building; otherwise, the structure may not be sound. Ultimately, you want visitors (the readers) to be able to construct a house for themselves with the materials that you supply, and it should look similar to if not the same as the house you have built. Not all suppliers will provide you with all the parts you need, however. It is incumbent upon you, therefore, to be aggressive about the acquisition of materials (i.e., finding all the information you need) and to identify structural weaknesses (**note areas of important missing or questionable information**). It is imperative that the visitor see all the key elements of the building and understand why they were put in. Also, it is important that you **thoughtfully *leave out* extraneous materials** from your building. They will only weaken your structure (and confuse your reader).

Make sure that, by the end of your write-up, your reader comprehends and can identify all the major and minor issues that you have neatly and logically organized. Two more perhaps obvious, but nonetheless important, aspects of communicating the H&P effectively are that **your language must be clear and understandable** and that **you must avoid making up abbreviations** that are not standardized and widely accepted.

✓ *Providing thorough background information about the patient*

Following the same metaphor, the background information is like the foundation of the building. The **more you**

understand about the history of the patient before the current problems arose, the better you will understand how the patient got to this point. That is, your house will stand more solidly, and you will have a sturdy base upon which to build it. Also, a solid foundation will help you predict future problems that are foreseeable and react to those that may not be. You will find that, once in the hospital, patients often develop problems that are unrelated to or, perhaps, only peripherally related to their primary presenting problem. Understanding their background may help shed light on any future problems that arise—with a solidly built house, you won't be left out in the cold. Doubtless the effort this requires pays off in your understanding of who the person you are treating is outside of his or her chief complaint.

> ✓ *Leading the reader through the information in an organized manner so he or she can understand what you were thinking when you made the decisions you made*

In some ways, the H&P can be a bit like a sales pitch. You give the reader as much of the information as you have deemed relevant and seamlessly guide the reader to reach the same conclusions you have made. The key here is that you have to **demonstrate your organizational and thinking processes.** This is probably the most difficult concept for the individual new to writing H&Ps. Your write-up must flow **logically (and often chronologically)** so the reader does not get lost.

"What is relevant?" "How do I organize it?" "Where does *this* piece of information belong?" The answers to these commonly asked questions are by no means straightforward. Hence, they are a source of enormous frustration for everyone new to this process—and **this is a process**. The only way to make it a less difficult one is to **practice and get critiqued** on your efforts. But remember, each critic will have his or her own bend on how to "build a house." Try not to take comments about style personally, but be sure to take comments about the substance and structure seriously. Over time you will develop your own style, which will, I hope, incorporate all three of the central aspects I mentioned in the first paragraph of the book.

✓ Sections of the H&P

Alright, enough of the theoretical mumbo-jumbo—let's write an H&P! One brief caveat, however, before beginning: **what follows is a general guide to writing an inpatient, internal medicine H&P**. Other settings (e.g., outpatient and intensive care unit [ICU]) and other specialties (e.g., pediatrics and surgery) will do this process somewhat differently. What does not change are the three central tenets discussed above.

Conventionally, the H&P is broken down into the following thirteen major sections:

1. Source
2. Chief complaint (CC)
3. History of the present illness (HPI)
4. Past medical history (PMH)
5. Medications (Meds)
6. Allergies (All)
7. Family history (FHx)
8. Social History (SHx)

9. Review of Systems (ROS)
10. Physical Exam (PE)
11. Laboratory and Data (Labs/Data)
12. Assessment/Impression/Summary
13. Plan

If you read various books or guides about the H&P, you will see that there are some slight variations to the above list in terms of order or in terms of the addition of other sections. I have pointed out some of these variations along the way.

Below, I go through each section, identify and explain its purpose, and give examples to illustrate it. Please note that, unless otherwise specified, each example is a brand new hypothetical patient and not one carried over from a prior section.

1. Source

The Source section of your H&P is a **very brief** statement **identifying where you got your information and how credible** you feel it is. This helps the reader understand how reliable your information is and explains why there may be different information included in various team member's H&Ps.

Example: Information obtained from the patient and his spouse, who seemed clear and coherent.

Example: Information obtained from 5-year-old son who acted as interpreter for the patient, who doesn't speak English. Son seemed to understand only part of questions.

Example: *Information obtained from drowsy, intoxicated patient and the police officer who brought her in, and it was supplemented by old medical records.*

2. Chief Complaint (CC)

This section is like a sneak preview of the house to be built. Typically, you will provide the following components: the patient's age, a brief but *relevant* past medical history, a few words (preferably the patient's words denoted by quotation marks) about what problem brings the patient to the hospital, and, finally, a statement about the duration of the current issue(s). This should all be completed in about two lines of text. Noting the race or ethnicity is often of debatable value, and many authors will leave it out unless it is epidemiologically relevant to the complaint.

Example: *34-year-old male with advanced AIDS complains of a "bad cough" and fevers developing over the last 8 days.*

Example: *81-year-old African-American female with a history of hypertension and diabetes complains of "pain in my chest" while walking up the stairs yesterday.*

Here I chose to include the race of the patient because responses to antihypertensive medications may vary between African Americans and Caucasian Americans.

Example: *56-year-old male with a history of ulcerative colitis complains of 3 months of worsening back stiffness, 2 weeks of "a sore on my leg," and 3 days of fevers and bloody, painless diarrhea.*

As you can see, these examples are the basics of the structure you are guiding your reader to build. You must include **just enough information** to whet the reader's appetite and to allow him or her to **begin focusing his or her attention on the major issues to be presented** in your history of the present illness.

Note, some authors will choose to make the Chief Complaint merely a few words that reflect exactly what the patient said: "I have a sore on my leg" or "I've been coughing up green phlegm for four days." This style is an acceptable alternative but requires that you incorporate some of the other information I've listed above into the early section of the History of the Present Illness (see below).

3. History of the Present Illness (HPI)

The HPI is one of the most, if not **the most, critical aspects of your H&P**. It reflects the fact that you took a thorough history, thought about it, and organized it for the reader. A clever student of mine explained that the key to writing (or presenting) a good HPI is **figuring out your assessment first**. That is, you have to think your way through the whole case all the way to the end, figure it out, and organize it *before* you write the HPI.

One of the keys to the HPI is understanding what information to include. Here, the answer is simple. Anything short of the current physical exam and laboratory findings that is *relevant* to the reason for presentation belongs in the HPI. Period. Ah, but how do you **understand what *is* relevant**? That is not simple, and it is where beginners at this process often run into trouble.

For example, if your patient has a cough with green sputum, the fact that he has a history of a bone marrow transplant **is relevant** because he will be immunocompromised and therefore at increased risk for infections. Another example: If your patient has abdominal pain, the fact that he has nausea and vomiting **is relevant**. So is the fact that he has a history of small bowel obstruction and is status post resection of small bowel last year complicated by adhesions.

These examples may seem obvious. What may not seem so obvious is that, in the first patient, the fact that he has a long history of smoking and has not had nausea, vomiting, diarrhea, dysuria, dyspnea, hemoptysis, ill contacts, bird exposure, or travel outside of the Boston area is also relevant. In the second case, it would also be important to include the fact that he has had poor oral intake and is dizzy but has not had syncope or presyncope. Also, you should note that he has not noted blood in his stool, had dysuria or polyuria, lost any weight, or been involved in any recent trauma. My point is that **you should include in your HPI *all* information—both pertinent positives *and* negatives—that helps shape your understanding** of the current issues. That is, these pertinent positives and negatives help navigate the reader through **the differential diagnosis** you considered.

It would *not* be important to include the fact that the first patient was recently started on new medication for hypertension or that the second person has a remote history of gout in the HPI. They do not contribute to your understanding of the current medical issues. Here is an example of a full HPI:

Example: M. T. is a 45-year-old homeless Vietnamese male who was in his usual state of health until approximately 5 weeks prior to admission when he began noting drenching night sweats occurring initially about 2 times weekly. The night sweats then increased in frequency, and about 3 weeks prior to admission, he also began having a cough. It was initially dry but progressed to being productive of small amounts yellow sputum tinged with blood. He also thinks he had fevers but had no access to a thermometer. He has been staying at various shelters around Boston. He noted that he'd been losing about 5 lbs/month without trying to diet and there had been no change in his activity level. This had been going on for about 3 months. He had no history of injection drug use, blood transfusion, or cigarette use and does not know his PPD status. He has had multiple sexual partners over the last few years he has been on the streets, including two experiences of trading unprotected sex with another male for alcohol. The patient admits to only sporadic condom use and says he forgets when he gets drunk, which happens a few times a week. He has not received either a flu or pneumococcal vaccine in the past though he had an uncomplicated admission in 2/97 to St. Elsewhere for community-acquired pneumonia. He stated that there were a lot of people at the shelters who had "colds" but didn't know any specifics about those illnesses. M.T. came to the USA about 10 years ago and has lived in Boston the entire time with no travel outside the city. At this time, he denies dyspnea, chest pain, nausea, vomiting, diarrhea, swollen lymph nodes, myalgias, arthralgias, decreased appetite, and rash.

A few points about this HPI: Note that I begin by telling you when the last time the patient was at his baseline. The initial statement that the patient **"was in his usual state of health until. . ."** gives the reader a time frame to use for reference. This information helps the reader understand **the chronology and chronicity** of the issues. The aim is for each line to allow the reader to generate and hone the differential diagnosis for the presentation in a logical and orderly fashion. Herein lies the central concept of the term *relevant*. **Anything that helps to fine-tune the differential diagnosis is relevant.** I included relevant information such as the PMH (his pneumonia in 2/97), habits (significant alcohol consumption and high-risk sexual activity), vaccines, and living situation—details that build **the context for the presentation**—and I ended with the so-called **pertinent positives and negatives.** You will see later that I will *not* repeat those findings in my review of systems. This information helps the reader decide among the aspects of the differential diagnosis (e.g., community-acquired pneumonia, tuberculosis, undiagnosed HIV disease with a related pneumonia, malignancy) and identifies the patient's **context** of what possible contributing problems (living in shelters) or comorbidities (substantial alcohol consumption) exist. The information also helps to identify particular risks to the patient's health (high risk for hepatitis, alcohol-related disease, HIV, and other STDs).

Remember also that the **HPI should be chock full of organized information but *not* analysis.** State the HPI without interpreting it here. (Do write: "The patient had burning on urination." Don't write: "The patient complains of symptoms consistent with a urinary tract infection.") Additionally, unlike other sections of the H&P, which may be written in short phrases or incomplete sentences, **the HPI should be written in full prose.**

The HPI is a **thoughtfully edited and (generally chronologically) organized summary of the relevant current information and previously obtained primary data** that leads the reader through the **differential diagnosis** of the patient's presentation toward the diagnosis (or group of diagnoses) that **you have already decided on in your assessment at the end.**

The Emergency Department Course

Where to describe events of the admission that occurred in the Emergency Department is an area of controversy. It would be prudent to find out the documentation culture at your institution. Some advocate including it like a minihospital course at the end of the HPI. They will include the exam and lab findings as well as any therapeutic interventions that have transpired and the patient's response. Others will only include truly remarkable findings on exam that have changed by the time the patient presents to the floor and will save lab results for the Labs/Data section below. Therapeutic interventions that had immediate results (e.g., nitroglycerin for chest pain or nebulizer treatments for asthma) may warrant mention because the response to therapy may influence the differential diagnosis and future management. Important but not impression-altering events (e.g., drawing blood cultures and initiating antibiotics) may be reserved for the Assessment and Plan.

<u>Note</u>: No diagnoses made in the Emergency Department should be listed in the HPI because they prematurely focus the reader's considerations of what is happening. That is, **identify facts, not impressions,** from the Emergency Department course. Make your own conclusions and diagnoses in the Assessment and Plan sections (described below).

Summary

A complete HPI includes the following **four components:**

✍ A **statement of the primary complaint(s) or issue(s)** that need to be addressed

✍ A **relevant context** for those issues, including previously obtained primary data, comorbid conditions, and any social situations, habits, or exposures that may contribute to your thinking about the presentation

✍ **Elucidation of the characteristics of the complaint** (e.g., duration, radiation, precipitating factors)

✍ **Pertinent positives and negatives** that round out your differential diagnosis

4. Past Medical History (PMH)

This section is generally self-explanatory. **It is a comprehensive listing of the medical issues the patient has had before.** Some authors segregate PMH from Past Surgical, Past Psychiatric, and Past Ob/Gyn histories. I will leave that to your discretion and that of the service you are working on. Keep in mind that being complete in this section is as important as in the HPI. Old records often are quite useful for filling in gaps here. **But beware! "Chart lore" is the affectionate medical colloquialism for errors carried through from H&P to H&P with no**

one taking the time to validate the findings. Imagine your embarrassment if you were to ask a patient about the history of "MS" (multiple sclerosis) that you found in her chart when it really should have read "M.I." (myocardial infarction) but had been misread six admissions ago by a tired intern and just recopied into subsequent charts. Believe me, this happens all too often.

Remember, during your training, you have the luxury of time that the housestaff may not. This provides you the opportunity to **be very thorough.** As a doctor, I always hope to find a compulsive student's H&P when I review a record because medical students can afford to spend the extra time needed to dig further and uncover *the primary data*. If there are primary data (e.g., CT reports, cardiac catheterization reports, pathology reports, pulmonary function test results, echo results), including them is useful. Also, when listing the PMH, it may be helpful to put it in chronologic order for events that occurred on a specific date (e.g., a test, event such as a stroke, or an operation). Diagnoses that are chronic (e.g., diabetes mellitus or chronic obstructive pulmonary disease) should probably be listed in order of importance or disease activity— although this is clearly subjective.

Example:

1. *Congestive heart failure. Last echo 4/01: moderate left ventricular hypertrophy. Left ventricular ejection fraction = 35%. Moderate MR/TR. New York Heart Assn class II 8/98. Seen in Heart Failure Clinic by Dr. Ven Trikel.*
2. *Type II Diabetes. Diagnosed 1993. Complicated by mild retinopathy (last seen by ophtho 9/98), and neuropathy in toes. Last urinalysis 2/03 negative for*

microalbuminuria. Checks own blood sugar 3x/week. Last HbA_{1c} 1/99 = 8.1.
3. Status post cholecystectomy 4/94 for gallstones.
4. Hypertension. Well controlled for 5 years.
5. Status post hysterectomy—details unknown—approx 1990 at Boston Hospital.

Example:

1. HIV+. Diagnosed 5/97. Treated with triple antiretro-viral therapy for the last 18 months. Last CD4 11/02 = 320. HIV viral load unavailable. Complicated by thrush and 1 episode of PCP 4/98.
2. Endocarditis of tricuspid valve 1995. Viridans strep. Attributed to IV heroin use. Echo 1/97: min TR otherwise normal study.
3. Injection drug use: Former heroin. Now in metha-done maintenance.
4. Melanoma on left thigh. 1988. Path: superficial spreading. 0.62 mm depth. Excised at BMC with 2 cm borders. No recurrence.
5. PPD+. Post 6 months INH therapy 1997.
6. Chickenpox as teenager complicated by pneumonia.
7. G3P2 SAb1

These examples illustrate the importance of being thorough and not listing just the disorder (e.g., congestive heart failure, hypertension) without further detail. Please note in this section, I would recommend **repeating things previously mentioned in the HPI as a point of reference.** For example, you may be presenting a patient with chest pain and wrote that he had a triple coronary artery bypass surgery in 1994 after an inferior MI complicated by heart block requiring pacemaker placement. I would still list in my PMH: "1. Coronary artery bypass surgery—see HPI. 2. MI—see HPI. 3. Pacemaker implanted—see HPI." This ensures that later on, someone who refers to your note for information on the PMH gets the whole picture. Yes, it is a bit redundant, but usefully so. This section need not be written in full sentences; fragments will do.

5. Medications (Meds)

The medication history includes **all current and recent medications**. It should also include **any over-the-counter medications and herbal preparations** the patient takes even occasionally. Also, try to include route of administration and the doses taken. If the dosing has changed recently, that fact should be noted. In most cases, it is irrelevant whether you use brand names or generics. A discussion of which medications require specification of the brand is beyond the scope of this book. Simply put, use the name of the medication supplied by the patient.

Example:
1. *Lisinopril 10 mg po qd*
2. *Lanoxin 0.125 mg po qd*
3. *Vitamin B_{12} 100 ug im q month*
4. *Pravastatin 40 mg (increased from 20 mg 3 weeks ago) po qhs*
5. *Multivitamin 1 po qd*
6. *St. John's wort (?dose) 1 tablet po qd prn depressed mood*

6. Allergies (All)

This section is one of the greatest sources of chart lore in the H&P. Patients often claim an allergy to a medication, and it is written in the chart without confirmation. When a thorough review of the "allergy" *is* made, one often finds that the medicine upset the patient's stomach or "didn't work for me" or had some other similarly nonallergic side effect. Therefore, **always confirm allergies yourself and ask what reaction patients had to the given medication**. (Additionally, find out if the patient has taken any other medication that is in the same class or family. This is often useful for identifying real allergy from a medication side effect. A classic example of this is a patient who claims to be allergic to penicillin but took amoxicillin without difficulty.) It is reasonable to include medication "intolerances" as long as you do not record them as "allergies."

Example: 1. *Sulfa drugs—rash*
               2. *Ampicillin—anaphylaxis*

Note: This is not the place for seasonal allergies, hay fever, or contact allergies. They belong in the PMH.

7. Family History (FHx)

The FHx is a bit of a misnomer, because the object in this section is to determine the family *medical* history. The importance of this information is that it helps **identify risk factors for certain diseases—either familial** (e.g., breast cancer) **or exposure related** (e.g., tuberculosis). Some authors advise that you actually draw out a family pedigree with circles and squares with lines indicating how individuals are related. This may be visually appealing. Others believe simply listing the close members of the family (siblings, children, parents, grandparents, and anyone else deemed particularly relevant) and any medical problems they may possess is adequate. Note if the patient says "my family is healthy," make sure you follow-up with specifics by asking "Is there any cancer, diabetes, heart disease, high blood pressure problems (etc.) in your family?" so that you can write the "pertinent negatives." Again, **if you believe the FHx is relevant to the HPI** (e.g., a father with a history of MI at age 43 is relevant to the patient's chest pain presentation), **it should be stated in both places**. This section may be written in prose, fragments, or simply with a pictorial representation of the pedigree with the appropriate diagnoses below the circle or square representing the family members.

Example: _Patient is youngest of 3 children. He has two older brothers, one 34 and the other 36. The 36-year-old was diagnosed last year with hypertension, and the 34-year-old has lupus and vitiligo. The patient's mother died in a car accident in 1996. She was presumed previously healthy. The patient's father has had a skin cancer removed (type unknown) and is treated for depression and anxiety. No information is available about grandparents. The patient denies a family history of diabetes, non-skin cancers, thyroid disease, myocardial infarctions, or strokes._

8. Social History (SHx)

Again, like the FHx, the SHx varies significantly among authors. Typically, the SHx will include information about the patient's occupation (including important exposures such as chemicals, dusts, radiation), personal interests, marital status, number of children, social support network, and living situation. Information about where the patient was raised and where he or she has lived previously may be useful to include as well. Habits such as smoking, alcohol, drugs, and sex should be discussed here, too. Whether you decide to lump them all together under SHx or split them up as SHx, Occupational History, and Habits is a point of personal style.

Example: The patient was employed as a meat packer during his 30s and 40s and recently left that to join his brother doing construction. He does lay insulation but has no known asbestos exposure and wears an industrial mask. His only chemical exposure is to paint thinner. He is married (22 years) and lives with his wife and three children in Chelsea in a single family home. He enjoys coaching Little League baseball and is taking a correspondence course to get his bachelor's degree. He denies cigarette use but admits to consuming 2–3 units of alcohol once or twice weekly with friends (CAGE questions 0 of 4). He denies illicit drug use and has had a monogamous sexual relationship with his wife since they have been married.

Example:

SHx:	*Married 22 years with 3 children*
	Taking correspondence course to get B.A.
	Coaches Little League baseball
Occ Hx:	*Does construction work (no asbestos exposure known)*
	Only chemical exposure is paint thinner
	Was previously a meat packer during his 30s and 40s
Habits:	*Denies tobacco and illicit drug use*
	Admits to 2–3 u alcohol twice weekly with friends

CAGE questions 0 of 4
Monogamous relationship with wife since
married

You will note that the second example here uses more truncated sentence structure. That is again a style issue. Generally, **it is preferable that the HPI, Assessment and Plan sections are written out in full sentences.** Also, if some aspect of the SHx is pursued in depth in the HPI, it merits only very brief comment here (e.g., I.V. heroin use—see HPI).

9. Review of Systems (ROS)

The ROS tends to be a quagmire of confusion for many students. Think of it as the attic of the house you are building. It is a great place to root around for interesting and potentially very important things, but it is not where you would place anything that could be more prominently placed somewhere else in the house. Simply stated, **the ROS is a comprehensive head-to-toe checklist to establish if the patient has any problems that are not directly related to the current complaints but merit further evaluation.** It is a fact-finding mission, but it always takes a backseat to the HPI. **Anything you find during the ROS that is actually a pertinent positive or negative for the current presentations belongs in the HPI, *not* the ROS.** Here, unlike the PMH, FHx, or SHx, you need *not* repeat things from the HPI. Any "issue" identified in this section will require further addressing in the Assessment and Plan sections (see below). Remember, things to include in the ROS are active or very recent problems, not things that happened in the remote past. The following is an example of an

ROS for the patient in the HPI section. Please reread that example (page 13) before proceeding to understand what I include here and, more importantly, what I intentionally do not repeat from that HPI.

Example:

General: *See HPI.*

Head: *No recent trauma. Occasional frontal headaches (1–3/month) with no associated symptoms of sinus drainage, jaw pain, visual changes, nausea, vomiting, or aura. Headaches relieved by Tylenol.*

Eyes: *No blurring, double vision, flashes/floaters, eye pain. Needs reading glasses.*

Ears: *No hearing loss, tinnitus, or ear pain.*

Nose: *No decreased smell, rhinorrhea, epistaxis.*

Throat: *No sore throat, odynophagia/dysphagia, abnormal taste, halitosis*

Neck: *No stiffness.*

Pulm: *See HPI.*

CV: *See HPI. Also, no palpitations, orthopnea, paroxysmal nocturnal dyspnea, or edema but does feel occasional "skipped beats" that last only a second and occur 2–3x/week. No Raynaud's.*

GI: *See HPI. No bloating, cramping, change in stool color/quality, or bright red blood per rectum. Positive heartburn exacerbated by alcohol and relieved usually by milk or antacids. Also, increasing mid-epigastric gnawing pain after eating over last few weeks, again, mildly improved by antacids.*

GU: *No dysuria, penile discharge, erectile or ejaculatory dysfunction.*

Musculoskeletal: *No joint pain except R knee from old sports injury. No swelling of joints, no muscle pain/weakness.*

Derm: See HPI.

Endocrine: No heat/cold intolerance. No recent changes in hat/glove size.

Psych: No depressed mood, sleep difficulties, or anxiety. He did note one episode about 6 weeks ago when he stopped drinking alcohol for a few days and began seeing bugs crawling on the walls that no one else saw. These stopped when he resumed drinking alcohol.

This is by no means intended to be an exhaustive ROS or the definitive style. There is as much inter-doctor variation on the questions asked and the format or categories used for writing up the ROS as there are variations in how people organize their attics. Nonetheless, the ROS should achieve the goal of fact finding in a useful way. For example, two issues that will need addressing later on in the Assessment and Plan are the patient's "heartburn" symptoms and his potential for alcohol withdrawal complications (because he hallucinated previously, he likely consumes substantial amounts of alcohol and may be at risk for withdrawal seizures).

Keep in mind, some suggest that issues such as "PPD status" (which is the screening test for tuberculosis) or "history of seasonal allergies" should be in the ROS. In my opinion, these types of historical issues more appropriately belong in the PMH or HPI because that is where most readers would look to find them.

10. Physical Examination (PE)

The physical exam should be viewed as the author's chance to demonstrate **physical evidence supporting or**

refuting the various aspects of the differential diagnosis that the preceding sections have suggested. Additionally, it should raise a picture in the reader's mind so he or she knows **what the patient looked like** at the time of your interview. This point should not be underestimated. As you will quickly discover when taking care of patients, the **"end-of-the-bed test"—that is, your gut reaction to how the patient looks** (does he or she appear acutely sick, chronically sick, basically healthy, about to stop breathing?)—**is extremely valuable**. Like many of the other sections, the PE style may vary from practitioner to practitioner. Try to adopt a reasonably standardized form (see example below) because readers will expect to find the information in a relatively standard order. Editorial comments and commonly used abbreviations are included in the following example in parentheses and using regular (nonitalic) type. Note that what follows is an example of an adult internal medicine physical. PE notes for other specialties may vary significantly. Also, sentences or fragments will do here.

Example:

General: *The patient appears cachectic, diaphoretic, in obvious respiratory distress, anxious, and older than his stated age.* (This is the "end-of-the-bed test." He looks sick!)

Vitals: *Temp = 100.6° F, HR = 144 (irr/irr—weak), BP 98/54 RR = 28 and labored.* (If you have vitals such as weight or oxygen saturation, they may be included here, too. Note that including the character and regularity of the pulse as well as the character of the breaths is useful. Irr/irr means irregularly irregular.)

Skin: *Moist without rashes, no tenting.*

HEENT (Head, eyes, ears, nose, throat): *Sclera anicteric.* PERRL (pupils equal, round, and reactive to light) *bilaterally. Swing test not performed.* EOMI (extra-ocular movements intact). (Strictly speaking this is part of the neurologic exam, but it is often included here.) *Funduscopic exam: normal disk and vessels bilaterally, but exam limited by patient's difficulty keeping eyes still. Tympanic membranes pearly and show a cone of light bilaterally with normal external canals. Nasal turbinates pink and there was no sinus tenderness. The* OP (oropharynx) *was moist with mild erythema of the tonsillar pillars without exudates or petechiae. Dentition normal.*

Neck: *Supple with shotty* NT (non-tender) *cervical* LAN (lymphadenopathy) *in the anterior cervical chain. There was no supraclavicular lymphadenopathy noted. The thyroid was normal.* (Organizational point: some will include information about the jugular veins and carotids here, whereas others will relegate that information to the cardiovascular section. Also, the lymph node exam may be listed as its own section or included as parts of other sections.)

Pulmonary: *Lung expansion is symmetric bilaterally. Auscultation reveals rales bilaterally about* $^2/_3$ *of the way up the back. There is egophony with decreased fremitus at both bases also. No wheezes or rhonchi noted. There is dullness to percussion at the* R>L *base.* (Generally, auscultation is recorded-before percussion in the write-up, but percussion is performed before auscultation in the physical exam. Why is this? Who knows!)

Cor or **CV** (cardiovascular): *The PMI* (point of maximal impulse) *was 4–5 cm in size, diffuse, and laterally displaced to the anterior axillary line. The heart beat was tachycardic and irr/irr* (irregularly irregular) *with an S_1, S_2, and S_3—difficult to hear with loud breathing. There were no m/c/r* (murmurs, clicks, or rubs). *The carotids were 1+ bilaterally without bruits and the JVP* (jugular venous pressure) *was estimated at 10 cm.* (Note, some authors choose to put the Cor section before the Pulmonary section. Also, the peripheral pulse exam may be included here by some physicians, whereas others will put it separately or under the Extremities section. Finally, try to write what you hear. If you think you heard an S_3 or a murmur, be bold and write it!)

(The breast exam often will be inserted here or just after the lung exam of the female patient, with comments about symmetry, texture, presence of masses, discharge, and tenderness, and abnormalities of the overlying skin. Breast exams on male patients should be done, especially if there is gynecomastia. Remember, 8–10% of breast cancers occur in men!)

Abd (abdomen): *The abdomen revealed normal active bowel sounds. It was ND* (non-distended) *but minimally tender in the RUQ* (right upper quadrant). *There was no rebound or guarding. The liver was palpated 3 fingerbreadths below the right costal margin at the midclavicular line and was smooth in texture. The spleen was not palpable.*

Rectal: *Exam revealed guaiac-negative brown stool with normal tone and prostate exam.* (Again, some will put the rectal exam as a part of the abdominal exam.)

Pelvic/GU: *Normal circumcised phallus with no masses or discharge and normally descended testicles.* (The female pelvic exam should include comments about the external genitalia, speculum exam, bimanual exam, and rectal exam, if not noted elsewhere.)

Extremities: *There was no evidence of clubbing or cyanosis. He had 2+ pitting of his LE (lower extremities) to the knees. Bilateral radial, brachial, and femoral pulses were 2+. The dorsalis pedis and anterior tibial pulses were difficult to palpate due to edema. There was no femoral, axillary, or epitrochlear lymphadenopathy noted.* (Again, the pulse and lymph node exams may go under a separate section heading if desired. This may be particularly prudent if an issue of the peripheral vascular system is central to the case.)

Musculoskeletal: *There was full range of motion of all joints in the upper and lower extremities except right hip flexion which was only 40° limited by the patient's complaints of pain in the popliteal area. There was evidence of thickening of the MCP (metacarpophalangeal) joints on all fingers of both hands. None were warm, red or tender. There was no evidence of joint effusions.*

Neurologic: *Cranial nerves (CN):*
> *I—not tested*
> *II—able to read newspaper print with reading glasses one eye at a time*
> *III, IV, and VI—extraocular movements intact*
> *V—facial light touch sensation normal*
> *VII—forehead wrinkles normally, no loss of facial folds*

VIII—patient able to hear whispers bilaterally at 3 inches

IX, X—palate raises symmetrically, gag reflex intact

XI—shoulder shrug strong bilaterally

XII—tongue protrudes without deviation

(Spelling out what you tested for each of the cranial nerves is wise, at least initially with a new preceptor, so you can demonstrate your understanding of the cranial nerves. Certainly any deficit should be explained explicitly.)

Sensory: *Light touch, pin prick, and proprioceptive sensation on the hands and feet were normal.*

Motor: (Here it is often preferable to make a chart of the muscle groups tested. Of note, some will do a similar chart comparing pulses right to left. The example [see table, next page] is obviously not a complete set of all muscle movements and groups . . . it's just all I could fit on the page! Additionally it is appropriate to comment on the patient's muscular tone and bulk.) *Tone seems normal throughout, but muscles appear diffusely atrophied.*

Deep tendon reflexes (DTRs): (For this section, it is preferable to chart your responses on a stick figure (see figure below), indicating the number grade of

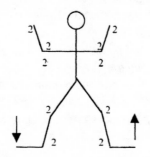

	Shoulder		Elbow		Wrist		Hand	Hip		Knee		Ankle	
	flex	ext	flex	ext	flex	ext	grasp	flex	ext	flex	ext	flex	ext
Right	5/5	5/5	5-/5	5-/5	5/5	5/5	5/5	5-/5	5/5	5/5	5/5	4+/5	4+/5
Left	5/5	5/5	5-/5	5-/5	5/5	5/5	5-/5	5-/5	5/5	5/5	5/5	4/5	4+/5

the reflex at the site of the tendon. Also, the plantar reflex may be denoted by an arrow showing the direction of the great toe's initial movement, up or down, or sideways if the patient's response was withdrawal or equivocal.

Coordination: *Finger-nose-finger, heel-to-shin, fine finger movements, and rapid alternating movements were all normal. Romberg testing was not performed.*

Gait: *The patient's gait was not tested due to breathlessness.* (Here, briefly comment on the characteristics of the gait, such as breadth of the base of the gait, the pattern of the gait, whether there is a direction toward which the patient leans, the speed.)

Mental status: *Due to breathlessness, formal mental status testing was deferred. He was, however, alert and oriented* (A&O) *to person, place, and date.* (This section should include some comments on how alert and oriented the patient seemed, at the very least. Additional comments about formal mental status testing, the Mini-Mental Status Exam, or other comments about mood, emotional tone, and/or thought processes may be included here.)

You may find some variation in the order of the presentation of the neurologic exam. It would be useful to find out what the local practices are in this case. To reiterate a point made earlier in the HPI: **report, don't interpret.** Document what you find on your exam, not what you think it represents. That comes later.

11. Laboratories/Data

At the beginning of your training, you need not worry too much about this section. It will become significantly more important once you are in a direct patient care role. As before, there is significant variability in the layout of this section. In general, **readers expect to see the "basic" labs first**. These generally include the basic chemistry labs (e.g., "electrolyte panel," "chem-7"), the complete blood count (CBC), liver function tests (LFTs), and coagulation studies early on; the more unusual tests follow. After the blood tests generally come the urine test (e.g., urinalysis [UA]). Subsequently, readers will look for the results of basic radiographic studies (e.g., the chest x-ray [CXR]) and finally the electrocardiogram (abbreviated ECG or EKG). Some authors will reverse the position of the chest x-ray and electrocardiogram. It is also often **helpful to the reader to highlight or circle abnormal values and to include normal ranges on tests that are less commonly ordered.** Also, remember to indicate on your radiology studies where you got your information (e.g., the formal report from the attending radiologist, a preliminary read by the resident, or your personal interpretation of the study).

You will also often encounter little stick figures that are used to facilitate lab reporting. The common three in use are listed here:

Chem 7

CBC

Coagulation Profile

Example:

$$
\frac{141 \;\;|\; 101 \;\;|\; 32}{4.1 \;\;|\; 32 \;\;|\; 1.5} \Big\rangle 77 \qquad 11.1 \Big\rangle\!\!\begin{array}{c}10.4\\ \\30.5\end{array}\!\!\Big\langle 121 \qquad \begin{array}{c}13.1\\ \\28.8\end{array}
$$

AST = **71** Ca = **11.7** PTH = **88** (normal 10-55pg/ml)
ALT = 24 Mg = 2.0
Bili = 1.2 Phos = 3.1
Alb = 3.0

UA: _Clear yellow. pH 6.0, specific gravity: 1.005. Trace protein. 1+ blood. Neg. nitrites/leukocyte esterase. 2-5 rbc/hpf_ (high power field). _0 wbc._

CXR _(per radiology resident in ER): No infiltrates, borderline cardiomegaly, no acute disease._

ECG: _NSR_ (normal sinus rhythm), _with normal axis and intervals. No acute ST or T wave abnormalities. No Q waves. There were no significant changes from an ECG from 2/96._ (Note, many computerized ECG machines will offer you an interpretation of the ECG tracing. Please try to ignore it! You should make an attempt to do your own interpretation. Besides, the machine regularly is _wrong_.)

The laboratory section is a place chock full of abbreviations that are difficult for the newcomer. Take your time learning them, and don't make up your own! This section is confusing enough.

12. Assessment/Impression/Summary

If I had my druthers, this section would *not* be referred
to as the Summary but rather as either the Assessment
or Impression (and note: the abbreviation "IMP" is
sometimes used for impression, but we *do not* abbreviate assessment!). The term *Summary* seems to imply a
regurgitation in short form of what has already been
said, whereas either of the other two terms tells the
reader "you are about to hear my brain working—these
are my thoughts." Here the reader must get the benefit
of your analytical powers, reading about how you tie the
case together and highlight all the key points. I will say
it again: **this is *not* simply a brief restatement of the
case. In fact, this section should not be brief at all.**
The sad truth is that a busy reader often will read only
your HPI and Assessment/Plan thoroughly and only skim
the rest. It must, therefore, **show all of your thinking
about the differential diagnosis and what data you
found to support or refute the various aspects of that
differential.** Note, however, that when presenting a differential, it is imperative to be thorough but not ridiculous. For example, if the patient is male, do not include
ectopic pregnancy on your differential diagnosis list for
abdominal pain; if your patient is bed bound and
dependent on a health care provider for oral intake, I
would not include water intoxication on the differential
of hyponatremia.

***Bad** Example: So in summary, the patient is a 46-year-old male with a history of Crohn's disease, hypertension, gout, left arm fracture, and is status post cholecystectomy who presents with complaints of 3 days of
fevers, abdominal bloating and pain, and blood-stained*

diarrhea. He is a truck driver and lives with his wife and one daughter. He uses heroin intranasally 2x/month. His exam revealed fever to 101 degrees, dry buccal mucosa and tongue, normal heart and lung exams, moderate right-sided abdominal tenderness with voluntary guarding, occult blood-positive stools, and normal cranial nerve exam. His labs show a white blood cell count of 13 and a hematocrit of 33. Other labs included a BUN of 34 and Cr of 1.6. The abdominal x-ray was unremarkable as were the ECG and UA.

A lot of good information is *summarized* above. In fact, starting this section with the words "so in summary" very effectively wakes up the reader and focuses his or her attention on the fact that something important is coming. What this example fails to do, however, is reveal that there was a sentient being on the other end of the pen writing it. Read what follows to understand this better.

Good *Example: So in summary, the patient is a 46-year-old male with a long history of difficult-to-control Crohn's disease who presents with complaints of 3 days of fevers, abdominal bloating and pain, and frequent bloody stools after tapering down his mesalamine dose. His exam revealed a mild fever, mild-moderate dehydration (orthostatic hypotension, dry mouth, flat jugular veins, contraction alkalosis, and prerenal azotemia), moderate right-sided abdominal tenderness with voluntary guarding, and occult blood-positive stools. His labs show an elevated white blood cell count and mild anemia. Notably, this presentation is similar to his prior Crohn's flares, and it seems most likely that this is a recurrence due to recent tapering of his maintenance medicine.*

Other possibilities include: infectious diarrhea (the patient's recent vacation in Mexico puts him at risk for agents like E. coli and Salmonella), appendicitis (with a trio of fever, elevated white blood count, and right lower quadrant pain), and incarcerated inguinal hernia (?small sliding hernia noted on exam—easily reduced). Less likely concerns would be: nephrolithiasis (The pain was not colicky and the UA shows no blood, but Crohn's patients are at increased risk for oxalate stones due to augmented GI uptake of oxalate from abnormal calcium absorption.), pancreatitis (The patient denies significant ethanol consumption, and gallstone-related disease is unlikely as he is status post cholecystectomy. Also, blood in stool generally is not seen with pancreatitis.), and herpes zoster (It is possible to have zoster without rash, but the distribution of the pain is not strictly dermatomal.)

Above, I have **reiterated the case's highlights and given my interpretation** of their meaning. I then carried the information to the next higher level: I developed a differential diagnosis and explained my thinking along the way. My **differential was then organized in order from the most likely to the least likely diagnosis, and I tried to offer an explanation for** *why* **the problem occurred** (he tapered his mesalamine).

If the patient has two or more major issues, as will often happen, you may find separating their assessments easier.

Example: In summary, this is a 59-year-old male with progressive shortness of breath on exertion with worsening edema in the lower extremities complicated by a purulent ulcerated skin lesion on his left lower leg. . . .

Here you might discuss the causes of the dyspnea on exertion and edema together, and then separately discuss the leg ulcer. Finally, you might try to tie the issues together, suggesting how or why they might be related.

13. The Plan

The end is in sight! To make your plan optimally effective, **keep it short** and to the point. **Enumerate your thoughts.** If your Assessment (above) is adequate, your Plan should simply flow off your pen logically, and little explanation should be required. Three organizational methods are commonly used for this section:

1. A specific problem list
2. An organ system list done in a set order
3. An organ system list ordered by relative importance

Each of the three has merits, and you should be facile with all so that you may pick the best one for your situation. The first method, the problem list, is created by listing the "title" of the problem and then writing a brief blurb about how you want to approach it. Many physicians consider this form to be the default, which suggests that it should be used unless there is a specific reason not to.

Problem List

When listing your title headings, **it is important to be as specific as possible here about what you think the exact problem is**. For example, it is preferable to write "microcytic anemia" over "anemia" because the former helps the reader understand why you are more concerned about iron studies and looking for hemoglobinopathies than the patient's B_{12} and folate levels. Remember, if you do not know specifics of the plan (e.g., what rate to suggest the IV fluids are to be run in a dehydrated patient or how frequently to give the nebulizer treatments to an asthmatic having an exacerbation), write a general statement indicating that you have thought about it (e.g., "begin IV fluids adequate to achieve rehydration" or "begin frequent nebulizer treatments"). Your supervisors should help you with those details. Additionally, **some topics you list may not have been addressed directly in your Assessment section, and, therefore, a brief statement of the problem may be required in the Plan section**. In the example above of a 46-year-old man with a Crohn's flare (see pages 36–37), my Assessment centered on the abdominal pain, glossing over the anemia, azotemia, and history of heroin use. These require *brief* commentary in the plan section instead of simply a plan.

Example:

1. ***Diffuse abdominal pain:***
   *Obtain CT abdomen looking for abscess or
       perforation.*
   *Stool for wbc (if +, will culture), and Ova &
       Parasites.*
   Will discuss with GI restarting patient's prednisone.
   *Begin IV fluids with potassium supplementation at
       250 ml/hr.*
   Consider oral metronidazole.
   *Ask surgery to evaluate patient if there is any
       deterioration.*
   Control pain with low doses of morphine.

2. ***Normocytic anemia:***

Likely due to anemia of chronic disease.

At risk for Fe, folate, B_{12} deficiency from Crohn's

   Will check Fe studies, folate, B_{12}, and blood smear

   No need for transfusion now

   Monitor Hb/Hct with rehydration—may fall

3. ***Azotemia, likely prerenal:***

Likely secondary to volume depletion due to

   increased stool volume and poor PO intake.

Will follow post hydration

No evidence of upper GI bleeding to raise BUN

May need renal ultrasound if not improved with fluids

4. ***Heroin use:***

At risk for progressing to IV heroin use

Possible candidate for Hep B vaccination

   Check Hep B panel

Will discuss with patient this high-risk behavior

Social work consult to address drug use

This format offers you specific headings and obvious problems to tackle. The limitation of this format is that it does not jog your memory about less central topics, such as the frequent headaches that you might have found in the ROS that you wanted to address. To avoid that problem, **it is often helpful to think through the second method (the organ system approach) in your head, even if you don't write it on your H&P.**

Organ System Approach

The organ system approach with a set order may seem cumbersome in many patients, but it **forces you to consider every organ system and address the issues** that arise. One order I occasionally use is: Neurology, Cardiovascular, Pulmonary, GI, Renal, Hematology, Infectious Disease, Endocrine, Rheumatology, Psychiatry, Social, Other. Feel free to create your own set order. The purpose is not to memorize *my* order but to create one for yourself that you can apply broadly and methodically to patients so that all systems get addressed. The more complicated the patient, the more useful I find this scheme. As above, however, it is crucial to elucidate the exact problem rather that simply relying on the organ section to substitute for the specifics. Again, for example, it is preferable to write "Heme: microcytic anemia" rather than simply "Heme" followed by your plan for evaluation.

Example:

Neuro: *Headaches likely tension related*
            Nothing to support migraine, subarachnoid
                hemorrhage, mass, cluster, or other
                ominous type of headache
            Tylenol as needed

CV: *Sinus tachycardia from pain, fever, dehydration*
            Aggressive IV rehydration
            Tylenol for fevers
            Low-dose morphine for pain

Pulm: *No active issues*

GI: *Likely Crohn's flare*
            Obtain abdominal CT looking for abscess,
                perforation, etc.
            Discuss with GI restarting patient's prednisone
            Surgery to evaluate patient if patient
                deteriorates
            Possible candidate for Hep B vaccination
            Check Hep B panel

Heme: Anemia, normocytic—likely "chronic disease"
   At risk for Fe, folate, B_{12} deficiency from
      Crohn's
      Will check Fe studies, folate, B_{12}, and blood
         smear
      No need for transfusion now
      Monitor Hb/Hct with rehydration—may fall
ID: Unlikely infectious diarrhea, but:
      Stool for wbc (if +, will culture), and Ova &
         Parasites
      Consider oral metronidazole for Crohn's
      Obtain blood cultures if temp > 101.5°
Endo: No active issues
Rheum: No active issues
Psych: No active issues
Social: Heroin user
      Needs aggressive counseling and
         intervention
      Social worker to assist counseling
      Will begin methadone to prevent withdrawal

You may feel this order is a bit contrived and artificial given that the main focus of this patient centers on his GI disease. In that case, you might consider trying an organ systems approach tailored to the patient's problems. I won't give an example of this style here other than to say you might organize it in the following order: GI, CV, ID, Heme, Neuro, Social, and then the rest in whatever order you want . . . or perhaps not at all. Here, too, **full prose may be used, although short phrases are often clearer**.

As above, **the Plan and Assessment sections may overlap** a bit. You'll notice, for example, that in the example above, under the Heme section, I do a bit of assessment of the anemia rather than just putting down a plan. Alternatively, one might opt to include the discussion of the anemia as an addition to the Assessment as a second issue. Be aware that if you try to do too many things in the Assessment you may find it becomes scattered and unfocused.

✓ Conclusion

The sheer length of this document should give you some idea about the complexity of writing up an H&P. It is difficult to do and even harder to do well. Do not get discouraged. Your learning curve will be steep if you keep in mind a few simple steps:

1. Remember the basic principles about the goals of the H&P listed on page 5. They will be important no matter what setting or specialty you are in.
2. Read over your H&Ps carefully before submitting them to the chart and your supervisor. Often your own proofreading can improve the quality of the H&P significantly, because you go from being the author to being the reader.
3. Insist on feedback on your H&Ps from your supervisors. This is critical to your improvement. Styles will vary from reader to reader, so don't get flustered by comments on style. Experiment with different styles until one feels right for you.

Good luck!

Writing a Daily Progress Note

Central to caring for patients is good communication. The progress note is the cornerstone of this process. Many of our patients require the participation of multiple services. The coordination of the plans and **understanding of the patient's needs require a combination of excellent written and verbal discussion**.

Writing notes is time-consuming and frankly can be onerous. It may seem that the time spent in documentation is taking away from the patient care. Learning the process of note writing well may tip you off to some of the benefits this skill affords both you and the patient. These benefits include:

- Organizing your thoughts
- Helping you identify areas you need to learn more about
- Making you rethink the previously made plans
- Reviewing the chart and others' written comments
- Ensuring you have addressed all the active issues
- Reviewing for errors or necessary changes to medications that the patient is currently receiving
- Documenting your efforts
- Helping you identify future problems that you may be able to preempt
- Getting you off your feet for a few minutes

There is no right way to write a daily progress note. What follows is an examination of the functional purpose of the necessary components of a note that will lead to effective communication. That is the primary goal. What follows are a few recommendations on the process of approaching the note.

✓ *The Approach*

Before setting pen to paper, **begin by reviewing the active medication list** kept by the nurses. If your system is computerized, the online list is the place to go. If you have a paper-based or combined computerized and paper-based system, use the system that nurses use to sign off on the medications once they are given. This way you know *exactly* what the patient has received. You should make this a habit daily or **at least every other day**. Trust me, you will find discrepancies and surprises.

Find the chart and preferably a quiet area to sit. Okay, at least a space to write! Begin **to review the chart going back at least as far as *your* last note**. Skim your note's Assessment and Plan and then thoroughly read any subsequent notes you have not already seen. Do not skip other services' notes because there is often valuable information there, too.

✓ *The Components*

This section is a discussion of the components of the note, *not* the order in which they "should" be presented. Comments on that topic will follow.

Date and Time

Make sure that you indicate the **date and time of your notes**. This not only is for legal purposes, but also helps future readers understand the chronology of events.

Identifiers

This term means two things. First, ensure that the paper on which you are writing has the **patient's name stamped** on it. If the name plate is lost or not available, legibly print the patient's name and medical record number in the addressograph box. Second, **identify what kind of note you will be writing**. This is usually done by indicating your level of training and the type of note being written (e.g., 3rd year medical student progress note [MSIIIPN]; intern progress note [IPN]).

Events

A brief **summary of any key events** that have occurred since the last progress note (e.g., chest pain episodes, hemodynamic instability, test results resulting in therapy changes), unless documented previously, should be included.

Subjective Statement

Here you will indicate what the main complaints of the patient were when you saw him or her. Like the Chief Complaint of a History and Physical (H&P), you may choose to **use either the patient's own words or your description** of the complaints. Unlike the Chief Complaint, however, this section should **include pertinent positives and negatives *strictly relevant* to the current complaint** and active problem list. In this way, it is like the History of Present Illness (HPI) section of the H&P. In addition to trying to elucidate new complaints, one should include comments on previous complaints, especially if there is a change, even if the patient does not volunteer this information without prompting.

Medication List

Make sure that you list the active medications daily or on alternating days (see comments above).

Physical Examination

Unlike your admission H&P, which should have been quite thorough, after the patient has been admitted you should move to a focused examination. This means that you should include the following:

- ✍ A statement about the **appearance** of the patient— especially if the patient appears unwell or the appearance has changed
- ✍ The **vital signs** (including the O_2 saturations, daily weight, and intake and output [I&Os])
- ✍ Comments about the exam of any part relevant to the patient's illness or current complaints (*note*: periodically a more thorough re-examination of the patient may be wise because the focused exam may overlook new findings)

Labs and Data

It is important that you **write in all labs and data** for which you have results and make note of those that are pending. Some lab tests take days or weeks to be reported. **Listing pending labs** will help remind you to continue to check if they have been reported yet. If a lab is pending at the time you are writing your note, make sure to write an addendum later with that information. When including data such as radiologic studies or pathology reports, be sure to write whether your report is preliminary or final.

Assessment and Plan

This section is truly the brains of your note. It may be disappointing for you to learn the truth, but many busy readers skip the above sections and go straight to this section when skimming a chart, so you must be thorough and clear here. The assessment section should begin with a *brief* **statement** about the patient and what seems to be going on with him or her. Remember, **it is not a regurgitation, it is a synthesis,** as with the assessment section of the H&P.

The meat of the assessment section is the listing of the issues. Two methods are generally accepted. The first, a **problem list approach,** is an organized, prioritized, issue-based compilation of the main areas of diagnostic evaluation, therapeutic intervention, or general concern. **Begin with the most important issue and name it as specifically as possible** (e.g., "acute-on-chronic pancreatitis," if that is what it is, rather than just "abdominal pain"). Remember to discuss changes in the status of this problem and any therapeutic or diagnostic options being considered, and enumerate your plan clearly. Then move to the next issue.

An alternate way to approach this section is via a **systems approach.** This method may be useful in intensive care unit (ICU) patients but may be used in non-ICU inpatients as well. Here, one **marches through the systems of the body and discusses the issues relevant to each**. One may choose to use the same order on all patients (e.g., Neuro, Cardiovascular, Pulmonary, Renal, GI, Heme, ID, Endocrine) for which the advantage is consistency and a forced review of systems you might not otherwise consider.

Others like the systems approach to begin with the most central or relevant system and address the lesser systems subsequently. Remember, the systems approach should not lead to diagnostic sloppiness or laziness. You must **still identify specific problems by name**. Your assessment should *not* read: "GI–Unchanged. Continue NPO with IM narcotics." It should say: "GI–Pancreatitis unchanged. Continue NPO with IM narcotics." Also, bear in mind that certain problems might not be classified easily using the systems approach. The classic example here is fever of unclear etiology. Do you put it under ID as a manifestation of an infection, under Rheumatology as a feature of an autoimmune disease, or under Oncology as a malignancy feature? The same issue occurs with other problems (e.g., hematuria, pulmonary infiltrates, chest pain), making the systems approach often cumbersome, confusing, and less precise.

When writing the plan, you may choose either to intercalate it into the problem list or system list (e.g., "Alcoholic pancreatitis: Improving PO tolerability and pain control. Will begin clear liquids today with continued pain medications as before") or list the plans after the problems. The latter style is useful if there is only one or a few issues that are closely interrelated. Otherwise, weaving the plan into the list of issues is preferable.

Signature

Make sure you sign all chart entries with **your signature, your name legibly printed underneath your signature, and your beeper number**. Additionally, students should try to seek out their supervisor to cosign his or her notes at or near the time the notes are put into the chart.

✓ The Order

The classic order of the above components is called the **SOAP note**, an acronym for subjective, objective, assessment, and plan. It essentially follows the exact order I have outlined in the last section. Be aware, however, that you will find variations that you may come across that are appealing. One alternative you may see begins with an event and problem list on the left margin and med list on the right margin. To the reader, this allows a foreshadowing of what is to come and what to look out for. The subjective, objective, assessment, and plan sections follow thereafter. An additional advantage here is that, by keeping a list of problems at the beginning, the reader can page through the notes and quickly identify the events and issues of the day. A third style, occasionally employed by more senior clinicians and *not* recommended for trainees, is a straight problem list approach. In this method, a problem is listed and discussed with the relevant complaints, physical exam, and lab findings noted, and the assessment and plan follow. One then moves on to the next problem.

The key is that the order is less important than the logic used to derive it and the thinking process it demonstrates. As long as the note flows in a reasonable manner, it is acceptable to deviate from the SOAP style. Nonetheless, it is preferable that students learn the SOAP style so they have that skill for other rotations that may require it.

✓ *Final Comments*

1. *Every day* that you see a patient, you should expect to write a progress note. It is encouraged that you write an addendum if additional information becomes available or the patient's status changes later in the day. This note may be abbreviated, but it is important.

2. Discharge day notes may be brief, but they are helpful so that others may understand where the patient went after discharge and in what condition, as well as what follow-up plans were made. The discharge paperwork that contains some of this information is not always available or clear so your note is useful.

3. Legibility is extremely important. If you are one of those individuals blessed with uninterpretable chicken scratch, your notes are worthless. Slow down. Print in capitals. Do whatever it takes to be legible. You will work too long and hard on your notes not to have them be readable.

Thanks for taking the time out to learn how to write a really good note. It helps your team, improves patient care, and is educational.

Index

Notes

Notes

Notes

Notes

Notes

Notes